N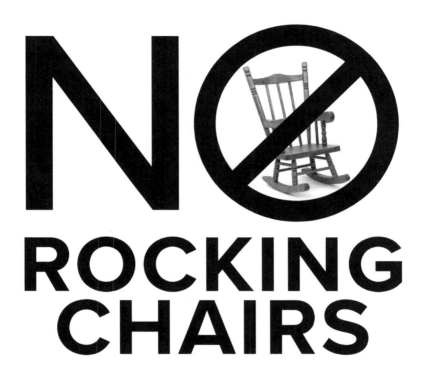
ROCKING
CHAIRS

HOW TO BE
PHYSICALLY MOBILE
AND ACTIVE
NOW AND IN RETIREMENT

Dr. Michael Kwast, DC, CSCS

No Rocking Chairs

ISBN (Print): 978-1-66781-583-1
ISBN (eBook): 978-1-66781-584-8

TABLE OF CONTENTS

About the Author 7

Introduction 9

The Ah-Ha Discovery 11

Reverse Engineer 19

Roadblock #1 Basing Health on Your Feelings 27

Roadblock #2 Excuses 39

Roadblock #3 Misunderstandings 55

So Now What Do You Do? 79

ABOUT THE AUTHOR

Dr. Michael Kwast is a graduate of Michigan State University and Cum Laude graduate from Palmer College of Chiropractic West in 1998. He was awarded the prestigious Clinical Excellence Award and is a Certified Strength and Conditioning Specialist. Since founding iChiro Clinics, the Clinic has been awarded the 2014 Better Business Bureau of West Michigan's Trust Award for Ethics, Grand Rapids Magazine's Best of Grand Rapids Chiropractor (2014, 2015, 2016, 2017, 2018, and 2020), Grand Rapids Chamber of Commerce Small Business of the year in 2016, and the Talk of the Town Award (2010, 2011, 2012, 2013, 2014, 2015, 2016, 2017, 2018, 2019, 2020, 2021). iChiro Clinics was established as a Pro Adjuster Center of Excellence in 2019. As a practitioner, and international speaker and author, Dr. Kwast has helped thousands of patients realize a higher level of health and function.

INTRODUCTION

"If you fail to plan, you are planning to fail."
Benjamin Franklin

E veryone knows planning for retirement is essential to have a good quality of life in their golden years. The 401k plans most people know about started in the late 1970's. People realized that Social Security was not sufficient to maintain the lifestyle they had grown accustomed to. Saving and investing was difficult and confusing for the average person, and people realized they needed help. Financial advisors became the "go to" people for advice and plans.

Today, most people consider retirement planning to be common knowledge and a "given" for many people in the workforce. There are numerous financial planners and advisors with numerous strategies and opportunities to plan and grow wealth for retirement.

Northwestern Mutual performed a survey and found in 2019 only 10% of respondents are confident that they have enough saved for retirement, and on average people said there was a 45% chance they would run out of money in retirement. Disturbingly, only 41% said that they have taken any action to address the issue.

While there are still plenty of people who don't plan properly financially, there is another problem of which many people are completely unaware. I would say this problem is even more disturbing than the financial issues described above. This problem destroys the point of retirement plans and fills people with regret, depression, and buyer's remorse.

This problem will be the focus of this book, and the problem is called a lack of Quality of Life.

THE AH-HA DISCOVERY

"It takes a wise man to learn from his mistakes, but an even wiser man to learn from others."

Zen Proverb

In 2004, I was sitting with my financial planner figuring out how to save the most for retirement. If you have ever gone through the process, most planners will do a data collection interview to find out all of your information and calculate what you will need financially to meet your retirement goals. Some of the questions planners ask are questions like these: How long do you expect to live? How much money do you think you will need in retirement? When do you want to retire? What financial goals do you have? What things do you want to do when you retire?

The last question started us on a very long conversation. I told him my dreams of golfing everyday, traveling the world, playing and spending time with grandkids, hiking mountains, and playing tennis. As we discussed, he brought up some very real frustrations he had as a planner. Because he knew I was a chiropractor and worked with patients' physical abilities, he explained an all too common occurrence he was witnessing.

His story went something like this: I have sat down with numerous clients over the years and conducted similar interviews like the one you and I just completed. What is exciting and fulfilling is helping clients reach their financial goals at retirement. I have celebrated with many clients at retirement parties as we would look at their funds and realize we had "done it." We had achieved financially the goals we had set, and that felt awesome.

What happened next, I did not expect. He then went on to explain that even though the clients had achieved their financial goals, there was something missing. What was missing was the reason for the financial goals. The WHY. Why did the clients delay gratification of spending money in the moment to be able to invest money to have it in retirement? Was it just to sit in a rocking chair and be able to pay bills, or, was it for something bigger? What was the WHY?

The WHY was the dream. The retirement dream. I can't wait till I retire so I can... Fill in the blank. What were they going to DO in retirement? No one says, "Sit in a rocking chair and be able to pay bills." Everyone had a list of activities and things to do such as travel, play sports, play with grandkids, etc. The interesting common denominator was the WHY was always something requiring a level of physical ability.

He then told me story after story of clients that had reached financial freedom in retirement, only to be disappointed and depressed because they could not actively participate in the dream. Their health and mobility was in such decline that they were unable to do any of the things they had discussed and put on the retirement dream board. The guy who wanted to golf everyday couldn't even play nine holes before his back was killing him. The lady who was going to travel the world couldn't even sit in an airplane seat for thirty minutes without being in pain. The woman who was going to play with her grandkids couldn't even get up from the floor. The man who was going to play tennis three times a week, couldn't even play at all with his bad shoulder. They ended up spending all of their retirement time and money trying to regain their mobility and function.

I had heard all these stories before from patients in my practice. They ended up spending their retirement time and financial resources trying to regain their physical abilities and health. Interestingly, so many of the problems we were treating in the office were problems that could have been prevented or minimized if the problems had been located and treated appropriately earlier. Most of the patients were full of remorse that they had not done something sooner to help themselves. They ended up utilizing short term temporary solutions with long term detrimental consequences of which they were completely unaware. They were sacrificing their health for wealth when they were young, only to then spend their wealth trying to regain their health.

Part of the confusion is how people define health. Most people think about diseases like diabetes, atherosclerosis, cancer, high cholesterol, or other illnesses. Typically, the word "health" doesn't create an image of physical abilities. Physical abilities are rarely screened or measured in today's healthcare system. Interestingly, physical abilities are one of the most important factors in having a good quality of life.

Spending your time and money in retirement to regain your physical abilities or health was not on anyone's retirement dream board. This is where buyer's remorse would set in. People were mad. They sacrificed and did without in their younger years by putting money aside for the future, only to spend it all trying to regain what was lost. Some of them died with millions of dollars in the bank that they never utilized.

I remember a patient telling me that he would have been better off spending all of his money when he was young and could do stuff, than saving it for retirement and not being able to do anything like he had done. He was full of regret. I asked him, "If you could still do stuff would your opinion be different?" He said, "Of course, the best would be to be able to retire and still be able to do all the things I have dreamed about." Quality of life.

My dad is a car guy. He always loved cars, and in his younger years spent all his money on them. I remember when I was a kid, and I would be riding around with my dad. He was always on the lookout for any cool cars. According to my Dad, the best cars were driven by "old, grey haired guys." My dad would explain how life wasn't fair. By the time you could afford an awesome car, you were too old to enjoy the car. Some of the old guys could barely get in and out of a low riding Corvette. My dad would say, "young guys should be driving around in the fast sports cars, and the old guys should be driving the station wagons."

All of these experiences started to click together. I thought, what if we could help people age better? What if we could find and locate physical problems and inabilities before they became a giant disaster? What if people could actually reach retirement successfully? Successfully, meaning being able to financially and PHYSICALLY do the things on their retirement dream board. This would create a better QUALITY OF LIFE for every person. Ah-Ha…

What is on your retirement dream board? One of the things I tell patients is, "I want to be 99 years old, feeling great and on the golf course, ripping drives down the middle at 250 yards, playing with my grandkids, and giving them hell that the old man just outdrove them. Then, I just drop dead into the sand trap." The idea of living a long, full, and active life is something I believe most people want.

I have had numerous opportunities to speak at local companies and organizations. I have spoken at several assisted living centers in Grand Rapids, Michigan. Here are a few of the things I have learned from interviewing residents: If they could safely live at home, they would rather be at home than the assisted living center. They would rather endure some discomfort and pain, if they were able to be independent at home. They would give everything they have monetarily, if they could have their mobility and function restored, so they could have the Quality of Life they wrote on their retirement dream board. Understand, these assisted living centers are very nice with many amenities. They have movies, dances, bars, games, pool tables, and excursions to sporting events and concerts. They do your laundry and have a restaurant for all meals and snacks, etc. In fact, I was kind of thinking it would be awesome to live there now. These are very nice facilities. The key is this: Do you have your independence? The residents I spoke with would still rather live at home and have their independence which is largely dependent upon their ability to move and function.

This ability to move and function translates directly into the person's Quality Of Life.

Unfortunately, many people don't know that there are things they can do that will increase their odds of achieving this high level Quality Of Life. There are also many things you can do to decrease your odds of success of achieving a high Quality Of Life. Most of the people I talk with believe mobility and health is just a function of luck and genetics. The good news is there is much more involved. Let's take a look.

REVERSE ENGINEER

"Begin with the end in mind."
Stephen R. Covey

U nfortunately, many people don't have a plan or goals for much of anything, let alone retirement. Certainly there is no plan for their functional mobilities and Quality Of Life. One of my first associate doctors used to say, some people are like a leaf in the wind just getting blown here and there with no control of what is happening and with no real plan of where they end up. Kind of sad when you think about it but all too common. It is easy to avoid responsibility for your choices when you don't feel like you had anything to do with what happens to you. You never really had any "choices";stuff just happens to you because of...Fill in the blank. This is the land of excuses and rationalizations for any and all poor outcomes. Not a very successful method in my opinion.

The next level plan after the "No Plan" is the "Hope and Pray Plan." This is where people just hope and pray that things will work out, and they will be where they want to be at some point. Action on their part is not required, in fact, they believe it is virtually useless. It is easy to adopt this type of planning, when you have not been trained how to set goals and plan effectively. If you have ever failed at things you planned, it is easy to fall into this category. It caters to people who don't want to be accountable or responsible for the consequences of their choices. Being accountable for your past choices is a very hard pill to swallow. Life is much easier if you feel like nothing is your fault. This holds true in all of life's endeavors, including your health and Quality Of Life in retirement.

I remember when I was in college and had a big exam coming up. It was hard to balance all of the fun things on campus and still study. I decided I would try the "Hope and Pray" method instead of studying. After all, I went to class and should be able to remember the material. And if God really wanted me to pass this test, God would give me all the right answers. Needless to say, I'm sure you can guess how the exam turned out. Luckily, I learned the lesson that hard work and effort are still important ingredients in successful actions. While hope and prayer are important and effective things to be doing, action is also required when planning out your future.

One of the best ways to determine the future is to plan for the future you envision. Reverse engineering is a great way to work backwards from what you are trying to accomplish. While you have probably already done this for the financial retirement plan with an advisor, it is also important to put together a physical retirement plan for the activities you want to accomplish in your retirement. Think about the things you love to do. What would your ideal scene look like on a day to day basis? Start with the very basics.

Imagine someone you know who is old. What are some of the things you see that they can and cannot do? There are many things that come to mind. When I watch older people I notice things that are important for anyone. Some examples are called Activities of Daily Living (ADL's). These are basic things you just need to be able to do in daily life. What are some of the Activities of Daily Living (ADL's) that are important to you?

Examples:

Get up and down from the floor

Get up from a chair

Walk

Climb up and down stairs

Tie your shoes

Take your shoes on and off

Take your socks on and off

Take clothes on and off

Wash/bath yourself

Use the toilet

Get in and out of the car

Drive

See blind spot in the car

Put key in lock and open door

Pick up mail from off the floor/ground

Make a meal

Do dishes

Do laundry

Make the bed

Prepare meals

These are all very basic level activities that you will need to be able to do in retirement for a good Quality Of Life. These are often ignored and just assumed to be activities you will be able to do without any problem when you are old. However, many people are in the assisted living center or nursing home because of their inability to do some of these basic things.

Now, make a list of higher level activities you would like to do in your retirement years.

Example:

Play Golf

Play Pickle-ball

Play Tennis

Walk

Wake surf

Hike

World Travel

Family Events

Garden

Mow Grass

These are the activities I want to be able to do in retirement:

1. _____

2. _____

3. _____

4. _____

5. _____

6. _____

7. _____

8. _____

9. _____

These are more along the lines of what most people think about when they make a list of things they want to do in retirement. It's the fun stuff. Why do you make a list? Especially a list of the most basic ADL's?

The first reason is if you have a plan and a goal, you are more likely to achieve the goal. I love to use the S.M.A.R.T. goal format. S=Specific. Make your goal very specific. M=Measurable. Make the goal measurable. A=Action. Make the goal something you can work towards. R=Realistic. The goal needs to be realistically achievable. T=Timely. The goal needs to have a time unit assigned.

S.M.A.R.T goals can be used for just about everything we do in life. By using this format, expectations are set which provides clear direction. My wife often uses this method. Sometimes I think it is all subconscious to her now, as she does it with everything. She asked me to do her a favor. She said, "On your way home, can you stop at the Family Fare Grocery Store and pick up ketchup, mustard, and eight hamburger buns and be home by 5:15pm?" The request is very specific, with measurable actions, and time that is realistic. The odds of me getting this done are already higher. A text message would increase the odds as well. Notice that I didn't say "guarantee" I would get it done. I could still easily blow it. However, these specific actions increase the odds of success, but nothing guarantees it will happen.

The second reason for setting these goals is to put them into your awareness. The part of your brain that is involved with filtering out unnecessary information and focusing on pertinent information, is called the Reticular Activating System (RAS).

I remember going to a networking meeting a few years ago. The realtor I was meeting with asked me if I knew anyone who was selling their house. I couldn't think of anyone. She then asked if I had seen any for sale by owner signs anywhere. I couldn't remember seeing any signs. We ended the meeting and I headed back the way I had come. On my drive home, I noticed five for sale by owner signs that were in peoples' yards. What was interesting is that I drove the same route to and from the meeting. So, I drove by those same signs on my way to the meeting, yet did not see them. It wasn't like the people ran out there and put all five signs up while I was having the hour long meeting. However, once the realtor put my attention on the idea of for sale by owner signs, my RAS kicked in, and I saw the signs on the way home. I was able to call her with five for sale by owners she could then contact. This is a real life example of how the RAS focuses your attention.

When it comes to these activities, you need goal setting. You also need your RAS to be laser focused on each and every activity. You need to be aware of where your level of function is with each activity. This will help you achieve the level of function you desire, and the retirement Quality Of Life you are looking to achieve. I will expand on these goals later. But first, let's look at some of the barriers you will encounter on your journey.

ROADBLOCK #1
BASING HEALTH ON
YOUR FEELINGS

"Symptoms are not enemies to be destroyed, but sacred messengers who encourage us to take better care of ourselves."
Food Matters

When I was a kid, I can remember my grandma giving my mom a hard time about taking us to the dentist. Grandma felt it was a waste of money taking kids to the dentist when their teeth didn't even hurt! Back in grandma's time, people didn't go to the dentist until they had tooth pain. Dentists spent most of their time pulling teeth. This symptom based mindset had poor long term outcomes. My great grandma lived with my grandma and grandpa, and every night there were three cups on the bathroom counter with their dentures soaking. I thought it was great fun to mix them up and wait for the morning. Back then, It seemed like every other commercial on television was a Polident dentures product commercial. Overtime, the dental industry figured out it was better to prevent tooth decay instead of just waiting for people to have symptoms and then pull teeth. Many dentists at the time thought that preventing the need to pull teeth would put the dentists out of business, so they resisted the movement. Once the Crest toothpaste commercials started appearing on the television, the mindset of the masses changed and preventing cavities prevailed. Virtually everyone today knows that you should see a dentist regularly to prevent problems.

Many people today still use the symptom based mindset when it comes to their physical bodies. Especially, when it comes to the musculoskeletal system. Aches and pains are minimized, and people think their pains are no big deal. Most treatments for aches and pains are simply symptom masking treatments with side effects. For example, Acetaminophen or Tylenol are commonly used to mask musculoskeletal pain, yet it is also the number one cause of acute liver failure (ALF) in the United States. So many patients I have treated over the last two decades had no idea the drug was just masking their pain and had side effects. They believed it was somehow magically fixing the problem.

Ibuprofen is another example. Many people don't realize that this has side effects, and some can be serious. Because it is an anti-inflammatory, people tend to take it for every little thing. They think it is safe, since it is available over the counter. They are also thinking that the problem is the inflammation, and not what is causing the inflammation. However, it can be easy to take too much, especially over time. Not to mention, masking the problem never really fixes the physical limitation.

What I have seen commonly happen in my clinic, is patients tend to take over the counter medications which just mask the pain. However, they think it is fixing the CAUSE. When I talk with patients, you can figure this out by asking them questions. For example, I ask, "What do you think the drug is doing?" Patient says, "fixing the problem!" Me, "What is the problem?" Patient, "The pain you idiot!" This is the root of the confusion. Patients tend to think the symptom is the problem, instead of thinking about what is causing the symptom. When it comes to most musculoskeletal problems, the cause of the pain is a strain of a muscle and/or tendon, and/or a sprain of a ligament. The cause is the damage to the soft tissue. While these types of injuries will heal over time, depending on the severity. When these tissues heal, they often heal with scar tissue, which creates more loss of motion, which creates a higher chance that the tissue will be injured again the next time the movement happens. The mechanoreceptors can also be damaged and then send inaccurate information to the brain. I have often witnessed this snowball rolling down the hill phenomenon. The patient gets hurt bending over to pick up a pencil. The cause of the injury was a tight restriction in their back that they didn't know they had. The tissue damaged was the muscles in the lower back. As these muscles overstretched and tore, the body responds with inflammation to help heal the tissue. The patient takes medications to mask the pain, and anti-inflammatories. The masking of the pain allows the patient to continue doing activities that further aggravate and injure the soft tissues more, but they don't feel it. The anti-inflammatories slow the healing process, making the injury take longer to heal. Typically, the patient will put heat on the area which increases even more inflammation. This cycle continues for a period of time which is dependent on severity and how much pain and discomfort the patient can endure. Sometimes weeks, months, years, the patient finally decides to go to the doctor and is usually given prescription pain medications, unless the problem has progressed to require surgery. If there is something surgical, they are referred for that procedure. Sometimes the patient will decide to come into my clinic, instead of going to get more medications. It is not uncommon that the patient has been on over the counter (OTC) medications on a regular basis for years.

I recently saw a patient with neck pain. She was suffering tremendously. She had tried prescriptions, but had too many side effects, so she stopped taking them and just stuck with the OTCs. Upon taking her history, she reported that she was taking about 30 Tylenol per day, for the past month, as the pain was worsening. She had no idea of the risks. She easily could have died from taking that much. She told me that she thought it was safe because her doctor told her to take it, and it was over the counter. Her history also revealed that the injury that caused this terrible pain was when she tried to reach into the back seat of her car while driving, and she "pulled" her neck. This is not the type of traumatic event that you would expect. Nevertheless, her Quality of Life was very poor. Thankfully, after a few months of proper rehabilitation, we were able to restore her function and mobility, eliminate her medications, and improve her Quality of Life.

I like to use automobile analogies because most people have an easier time understanding. Imagine if your car was making a weird squeaky noise as you drove down the road. The noise, or symptom was getting louder as you drove around. You decide you should take it to the mechanic. As you drive up to the mechanic shop, he hears you coming. You pull up and explain the situation. He listens intently, and says that he can hear the noise. He then says, "I can fix it". He reaches inside the car and grabs the knob on the radio. He precedes to turn up the radio so loud that you can no longer hear the disturbing squeaking noise. With a smile on his face, he looks at you and says, "There, it is fixed". Would you be satisfied with that level of service from your mechanic? How about your doctor?

This symptom masking approach has led to many disasters. As you mask symptoms, the underlying cause of the problem typically gets worse, requiring more and more symptom masking. One pill turns into two, then five, then 10, then 20 then... We have recently witnessed this approach causing the opioid epidemic in the US. Sadly, many people have died, and many more have had their lives destroyed all because the concept of masking is not fixing was not clearly understood, even by healthcare providers.

I have volunteered at a homeless shelter in my town for more than 10 years. The shelter has a bunch of free services they offer to the people they serve. One of the services is free chiropractic care. Virtually all of the patients I have treated there were addicted to drugs. The drug addiction is what led to their situation of homelessness, despair, and life ruining situations. Many people in my town have the perception that the drug addicts at the shelter are there because they were big party people, or spent time on the Ozzy tour bus. However, that is not the case. The interesting part is when I took a history, the vast majority of the patients started their drug problem with a minor ache or pain. When they then self treated with OTCs, or were prescribed pain medications by their doctor, they went down the snowball hill. Two pills became, four, then 8, then 12, then addiction… What is great about the free clinic is that we are able to educate and treat patients without medications. We can treat the cause of the symptom and help them, so they can get back on their feet and have a better Quality of Life.

Realize, that pain is the body's way of communicating that something is wrong. You need to stop doing what you are doing. When this message is masked, the odds of further injury goes up. I was working with the owner of a company who was frustrated by the number of workers' compensation claims they had that turned into long term disability claims. I asked him to give me a typical scenario. He described it as follows: When an employee would hurt themselves lifting or doing something physical, we would send them to the company doctor. Generally, the doctor would give the employee a prescription, and a couple of weeks on the couch. The employee would come back to work two weeks later, feeling fine. Within a short time the employee would be injured again, usually the same body area was re-injured. The medications continued, and the length of time on the couch would increase. Eventually, the employee would be permanently off work, on workers' compensation and disability. This is a very expensive and ineffective approach based on masking symptoms, while ignoring the cause of the problem in the musculoskeletal system. Think about if you did that with your car... Just turn the radio up loud... Then just put the car in the garage and hope it will be better... Not fixing the problem.

Clearly, there is a time and place for everything. If someone is dying, perhaps masking their pain would be a good idea so they can pass in peace. After a traumatic accident, masking the pain would probably be a good idea as well. I am not advocating that medications should never be used. However, I am suggesting that they are used too frequently and inappropriately with very detrimental effects to the patients.

If it is a bad idea to base how you are doing, on how you feel, what should you do? The answer is easy. What do you do with everything else? Testing. Do you get check ups at the dentist? Or wait till your teeth hurt? Ladies, do you get a routine mammogram, pap smear, and bone density test? Or wait till you are hurting and having symptoms? Guys, do you routinely get a blood pressure check, prostate exam, and colonoscopy? Or, wait till you have symptoms? What is better, to do tests early or wait till there are symptoms?

Think about this, what if you went to the dentist and said to just look at the third tooth back on the top right side because that was the one that hurt. As he looked at the rotten tooth, he saw four other areas of developing decay. What would you want him to do? Just work on the symptomatic tooth, or address the asymptomatic teeth too? Would the dentist be doing you a service or a dis-service by only working on the symptomatic tooth? Would you say how great the dentist was because he only treated the symptomatic tooth? Would you compliment the dentist about how you weren't over-treated or "sold" to work on teeth that didn't even hurt? Or, would you be furious that the dentist allowed a small minor problem to turn into a giant future problem?

What if your medical doctor found something on a lab test, but you didn't have symptoms? Would it be a "sales pitch" for you to start taking actions to help with your asymptomatic condition? Would you think that was a rip off and scam? Or would you be grateful and thankful?

Why are people not doing physical ability testing? When it comes to physical abilities, I have observed most people just don't know that there are even physical ability tests available. This includes people in healthcare too. That would be like not knowing there were medical or dental tests to determine how your asymptomatic body was functioning. In my office, we always test a patient's physical abilities, so we can then retest later to ensure we are making progress. In my experience, there are very few patients who understand physical assessment testing, and even fewer who understand the ramifications of ignoring those findings. Sadly, the same holds true for many healthcare providers.

One of the technology breakthroughs in the Chiropractic profession is the Pro Adjuster. This technology is capable of measuring the motion of each individual vertebrae via a scan with a piezoelectric sensor. The technology is able to then treat the area of decreased and improper motion via a stretch reflex stimulation to the mechanoreceptors in the muscles around the vertebrae. By restoring the motion, relaxing the muscles, and improving the mechanoreceptors function, the patient not only functions better, but is able to feel better too. One of the huge benefits of this technology is measuring the motion. This means you can assess the patient's mobility, without relying on the patient's symptoms or feelings. We can then detect areas of poor function and mobility prior to the injury occurring. This technology is an important tool that allows you to measure joint motion. The ability to measure the joint motion before and after each treatment ensures you are making progress each time. I believe this technology is groundbreaking for the Chiropractic profession, and for patients globally. To be able to measure and test joints is critical for ensuring patients remain mobile and active in retirement. I personally have taken and demonstrated this technology to over one hundred medical clinics in Grand Rapids, Michigan. Guess how many medical doctors were aware of the technology? The answer was none. Not one. Sadly, these same doctors are the ones recommending what treatments patients should choose. Hard for them to make good recommendations when they are not even aware of the options.

Imagine if you had a great rotary phone. One like from the 1980's. If you never kept up and learned about new technologies, you would still be using that rotary phone today. The amazing smartphones of today would be unknown. Most of us wouldn't be able to survive without today's smartphone. It is essential that healthcare providers are kept up to date on all the new technologies and strategies available for their patients to have the best outcomes. It is equally valuable for the public to be aware of the options available in healthcare. Most people are not aware, and then often make very high risk choices that can have poor outcomes. I believe that people should be informed and have access to the choices available. I also believe that there should not be financial discrimination based on the patient's choice. For example, to have a knee joint replacement which costs the patient nothing, versus 3 months of therapy that end up costing thousands of dollars. Which would you pick if you didn't have any money? There is currently an unequal playing field in the insurance world that forces patients to make choices based on costs.

There are also many physical ability tests that are available. Some of the most common are: Range of Motion testing, Orthopedic testing, and Palpation testing. These tests can be very useful to find areas of increased risk of injury, the cause of chronic pain and dysfunction, and the cause of accelerated degeneration and arthritis. By utilizing these tests, you can ensure your joints are moving effectively, to give you better odds of success in reaching retirement with good function and mobility, which results in a better Quality of Life. However, you have to rely on the testing, and not just how you feel.

"Ok, so what do people do?" Don't panic, I'm getting there. First, let's look at some more roadblocks to that goal of a retirement that is active with a great Quality of Life.

ROADBLOCK #2
EXCUSES

"You can have your results or excuses, not both."
Arnold Schwarzenegger

I ndividual responsibility and accountability seem to be difficult for more and more people these days. Rationalizations and justifications are the norm. I have been observing this trend socially, as well as in healthcare. People like to have someone or something to blame. This somehow absolves them of any responsibility for the situation they are experiencing. This makes people feel better about themselves. Many people seem to want to be perceived as an innocent bystander in life, then they get hit by the bus of bad luck circumstances, with consequences that are unjustly forced upon them. The reality is that we can control numerous things that impact our odds of ending up with a high functioning Quality of Life in retirement.

One common excuse is AGE. People will say, "I'm just getting old". Many people want to blame their problems on age. After all, you can't do anything about age. This absolves the person from any responsibility from what they are experiencing. I have had 25 year old patients tell me that their back pain is because they are "getting old".

Now, I am not saying that age doesn't play a part in people's health. It certainly does. However, think about it like this: What if I bought two brand new corvettes when I was 16 years old. One was red and one was green. I Drove them both everyday on the exact same road, for the exact same time, at the exact same speed, put the exact same premium gas in them, washed them exactly the same, all the variables were the same. However, the red corvette would only get an oil change when the oil light came on, and would only get any kind of maintenance when there was a symptom. I would only rotate tires when the car started to shake. I would only check the air pressure when the car would seem lopsided. I would only put new spark plugs or get a tune up, when the car's engine showed me a symptom.

Now the green corvette was another story. I would get routine oil changes and maintenance. I would test and check the oil, the fluids, air pressure and other things regularly. Now ask yourself, which car do you think would last longer?

Obviously, the green corvette would last longer because I was taking better care of the vehicle. The same holds true with your body. The better you take care of your body along the way, the better your body will last. The better you take care of your body, the higher your Odds of Success will be at living a retirement with a high functioning Quality of Life.

Another common condition that is blamed on age is osteo-arthritis or degenerative joint disease (DJD), and degenerative disc disease. These are the arthritis's most people are talking about when they mention arthritis from old age.

I had a guy come into the clinic back in 2000. He came in and explained that his hip was "shot" and the medical doctor wanted to replace his hip, but he wanted to get my opinion. I agreed to take a look. While taking his history, I asked him what the medical doctor had told him. He said, "The dr. said my hip is worn out and needs to be replaced". I asked, "Did the doctor tell you WHY it was worn out and needed to be replaced?" He looked at me confused, and said, "Because I am old!" I said, "Ok, let me look at the chart. Yup, I exclaimed, you are old, you are 74 years old." He looked at me with a look of satisfaction. I then asked him, "How is your other hip?" He said, "There is nothing wrong with that one, it is fine!" I then asked, "How old is that one?" He sat silently for a long time, then said, "Good point." Think about it like this, if arthritis was caused from age, then every joint in your body would be worn out exactly the same. Every joint from your little toe, to your knee, to your hip, to your back, to your neck, to your shoulder, to your little fingers. All of them would be worn the same. What is interesting, is that you never see this in practice. There are always certain joints that are worn out more in certain people.

So what is the cause if it is not age? Here is the missing component. The muscles. When muscles are injured or strained, even subtlety, the muscle will tighten and shorten. This tightening will compress the joint, putting excessive compressive forces on the soft tissues and cartilage inside the joint. The muscles around every joint can cause compression in the joint, which then causes the joint to wear out at a faster rate. So the formula is: joint compression + time= arthritis. The longer a joint is compressed, the faster it will wear out. What is compressing? The muscles around the joint. The bone will even remodel to the stresses the muscles are causing. This is called Wolfe's Law.

You can even see patterns in people who do certain activities frequently. For example, frequent golfers tend to have more arthritis in the lower back and hips. Data entry workers tend to have more degeneration in their neck, wrists, hands, and fingers. Hair stylists tend to have more arthritis in their hands and fingers. Baseball pitchers tend to have more arthritis in their pitching shoulder. If the muscles around the joint have a high likelihood of being strained regularly, you have a higher chance of arthritis. If you mask the muscle pain, you will likely make it progress faster and be more severe.

Imagine you just bought 4 new tires on your corvette. You are busy driving around town, squealing the tires and jamming your music. One day you stop to get premium gas, and you notice that one of the tires looks funny. You walk over and take a look and notice abnormal wear on the outside of the front left tire. The car is working fine, and has NO symptoms, however, you noticed the tire looked funny. You decide that you should take the car back to the tire shop and show them what you found. When you get there, the mechanic takes a look and exclaims, "I know what the problem is!" "What is it?" you ask. "You have an old tire!" he explains. You ask, "What do you mean, an old tire?" He says, "Yeah, see how it is worn out from being old." You argue, "But I just bought all 4 tires at the same time and they are the same age, why is this one worn out faster than the other three?' The mechanic says, "It is because it is old." What would you say? What would you do? I would probably throw the tire through the window of the shop like the old Discount Tire commercial. You would never accept this explanation from your mechanic. Most of us know abnormal tire wear can come from the car being out of alignment. The system puts too much pressure on one tire, and causes the tire to wear out prematurely. Why do you accept this explanation for your joints from your doctor?

Remember the minor sprains we talked about earlier? These muscles get hurt from things we do in life, and the muscle tightens and shortens. What do you think happens if the muscles that are tight and short cross over a joint? Correct, the joint will be compressed. This compression puts excessive wear on the tissues and cartilage in the joint, causing the joint to wear out faster than it should.

The short tight muscles are compressing the joint, what do you think would happen if you just masked the pain? Can you see that you would allow the compression to worsen? As your body screamed in pain to your brain that the joint was being compressed, you had the music too loud, and couldn't hear it. A recipe for joint degeneration, prescription drug addiction, and likely joint replacement.

"I'm getting a NEW hip," is something I have heard many times over the years. If not a hip, a knee, a shoulder are the common joints replaced. Patients get very excited about the idea of having a "new" joint. After talking with numerous patients, I discovered a major misunderstanding. The "new" joint they were going to get, in their mind, was a joint that functions like it did when they were young. Meaning, they were going to be able to do all the things they did when they were young. After all, it is a "new" joint.

While many joint replacements are completely necessary, the expectations patients have are often totally unrealistic. The "new" joint doesn't move like they thought it was going to move. Often, the joint pain is relieved with the replacement, however, many times the disability remains on some level. Restrictions in weight and certain movements go along with the surgery. Not the "new" joint the patient thought it was going to be. Odds of better mobility are higher if the patient does proper rehabilitation after the replacement, however, few patients seem to follow through as it can be difficult, painful, and time consuming. It is also interesting to note, most joint replacements need to be redone after 10-15 years. Think about that for a moment. Why would a "new" joint made out of metal and plastic wear out so fast? You would think metal and plastic would last longer than bone?

Imagine my car example again. You are driving around in your corvette, and you notice one of the tires seems to be more worn. You head over to the mechanic shop, and show them the tire. They say, "Yup, it's all worn out." "Guess we will put a new one on." If they just put a new tire on, what would happen to that new tire over time? The tire would wear out again, faster than the older tires. Why? The cause of the abnormal wear was not addressed. The tire was just replaced. No one bothered to look at the reason why the tire was wearing out excessively. The reason for the excessive wear is that the car is out of alignment, and putting too much pressure into the tire, forcing it to wear out faster.

When you simply replace a joint in the body with a "new" metal and plastic joint, but don't address why the joint wore out in the first place, what do you think will happen? Most people don't even think about this situation. If the muscle imbalances that caused the abnormal joint compression are left unchanged, the new joint will obviously wear out too. The more compression and dysfunction, the faster the joint will wear out.

One of my patients was an avid outdoorsman. He liked to travel the world and hike around hunting and fishing. He had a "bad" knee from playing football in high school and college, and was always told that one day he would need to get it replaced. While he had several scopes of the knee over the years, he never did any rehab of the muscles. While he could get around very well for his age, his knee would bother him with aches and pains. One day the doctor talked him into getting it replaced, since his insurance deductible was already met, that would save him thousands of dollars. He ended up having a knee replacement. The surgery was a success, and after several months of healing, his pain was much less. This was great. The problem was, his knee didn't function like the old, injured knee. He couldn't hike for more than a few hundred yards. He couldn't climb mountains or even small hills. His balance was now much worse. While I recommended therapy, he just wouldn't do it. He now has less knee pain, but he also can't do the things he loved to do. All his activities are limited. Not the Quality of Life he envisioned with his "new" knee. Certainly not the active retirement he wanted.

The dreaded hunchback posture is something you see every-day. Often, people just attribute the elderly hunchback with compressions fractures. After all, you can't do anything about that, right? Most hunchback postures are not from compression fractures. They are simply from years of bad posture, adding up like straw on the camel's back. Overtime, you get a nice hunch. So the excuse is age, right? Even younger people are getting the hunch as they sit looking at their phones and tablets for hours on end. What do you do about it, besides working on posture? Fortunately, there are many therapies that can reverse this posture over time. Intersegmental traction combined with the Pro Adjuster posture protocol are great tools. While you may not see the same posture as you had when you were 18, I have always seen some level of improvement in every patient that was treated.

A 68 year old guy was coming into my office for low back pain. After our evaluation, I found several other asymptomatic problems. One of the concerns was his hunchback posture. On his intake form, he stated that he was 6'6". When I would talk to him, he looked me straight in the eye because of his hunch, and I am only 6'1". After about four months of therapy, and measurable improvements in his symptoms, and functional testing, he went for a regular check up at his medical doctor's office. The last checkup they measured him at 6"0". This check up he was measured at 6'6"! The nurses were confused and thought they may have just written it wrong on the last measurement. He went on to explain that he had been going to the chiropractor. The nurses joked saying that the chiropractor must be making you grow. While I wasn't making him grow, I was helping him to reverse his hunchback posture. He was standing taller. One of the first things people use to determine your age is often posture. So, he was looking "younger," and standing taller. Another thing people don't tend to consider is your odds of falling. If you are hunched forward, you are already the leaning tower of Pisa. It doesn't take much to send you falling forward, when you are already part way there. I would say he probably reduced his chances of falling by standing taller. This is a big deal, as falls are one of the top reasons that people end up going to live in a nursing home. Again, not something that is on anyone's retirement dream board.

Another excuse is LUCK. Some people think that life is just a function of luck and chance. If you get arthritis, it is just luck. If you get diabetes, it is just luck. If you have a heart attack, it is just luck. If you are inflexible, it is just luck. While luck and chance are always at work, I believe there are things that you can do to set the odds at the table you are playing.

I am not much of a gambler, however, I have seen people betting on sports and playing games of chance. When you are betting on the horses, there are certain odds that each horse has of winning based on a bunch of factors. These factors determine the odds. When it comes to a person reaching retirement, with good function, so they have a good Quality of Life, there are certain factors that determine the Odds of Success.

Imagine we clone you. You #1 eats healthy, takes vitamins, exercises regularly, manages his stress, keeps a healthy weight, drinks water, avoids smoking, avoids alcohol, gets routine medical massages, takes no over the counter medications, needs no prescriptions, gets routine checkups at the dentist, MD, and chiropractor.

You #2 eats fast food, doesn't exercise, is overweight, smokes, drinks excessively, takes over the counter medications weekly, takes several prescriptions, doesn't bother to see the dentist or chiropractor, and basically just gets refills on prescriptions at his MD's office.

As you can see, You #1 is setting the odds for his Quality of Life by working on the factors that make a difference. You #2 is also setting the odds for his Quality of life by not working on the factors that make a difference. What is cool, is you get to decide on your Odds of Success by what actions you decide to take.

Another excuse is Genetics. Some of the things I have heard in the clinic over the years are:

"My dad had a bad knee, too."

"Back pain runs in my family."

"Arthritis runs in the family."

"No one runs in my family." LOL

"No one in my family can touch their toes."

It is like you are doomed to experience the same thing as your ancestors and there is nothing you can do about it at all.

Genetics are another thing people like to use to eliminate their responsibility. After all, you can't change your genes. Or can you?

There is a lot of emerging research in the field of epigenetics. Epigenetics is the study of how your behaviors and environment can cause changes that affect the way your genes work. Epigenetic mechanisms do not change the DNA, however, change the way the DNA is read or expressed. Certain lifestyle factors have been identified that can potentially change your epigenetic patterns such as diet, obesity, physical activity levels, smoking, alcohol consumption, and working nights. Notice that these are things you can do to change your Odds of Success. That is no coincidence.

In a nutshell, what researchers are finding is that identical twins (same DNA), can have very different health outcomes. One twin has cancer, the other does not. One twin has diabetes, the other does not. One twin is obese, the other is not. One is flexible, the other is not. Remember, these are people who have the same DNA. So how can they be different? I thought we were at the mercy of our genes? Well, the epigenetic mechanisms can turn the expression of these genes on and off. What makes the epigenetic mechanisms turn genes on and off? Lifestyle. So you have more control than you think. In fact, when the identical twins' genes are compared in later life, there are many changes that have occurred in the epigenome and how their genes are being expressed. They don't look the same, because lifestyle has caused genes to be turned on and off.

Take identical twins Bob and John. Bob does very healthy things. He exercises, eats healthy, utilizes dental and chiropractic care preventatively, avoids drugs, doesn't smoke, avoids alcohol, drinks water, and takes vitamins. John eats junk food, smokes, takes numerous medications, drinks soda instead of water, doesn't exercise, doesn't go to the doctor unless he is hurting or having a symptom. Can you see how what you do can make a difference in how your DNA is expressed via epigenetic changes via lifestyle choices? This is astonishing. While this gives people a disturbing amount of responsibility, this should also give people hope to all those who think they are stuck in a place of bad health because of their genetics.

Another excuse is thinking that what you do will not matter.

I have witnessed so many patients over the years fall into these traps. Because they think their problem is age, genes, or inevitable consequences from past injuries, people fail to act.

A friend of mine had injured her knees when she was young. She had major surgeries to repair what could be done, however, her knees would never be "normal". The doctors told her that she would eventually need bilateral knee replacement. Because she was told this, she believes that there is nothing she can do to influence her situation. She believes she is inevitably doomed to an eventual knee replacement. She may be. However, what if she could take actions that would buy her more time before she needed the knee replacements? What if she could buy enough time, that she ended up not needing the knee replacements? These are all questions to ask and consider, as surgeries are not without risks. In fact, surgeries are considered a last resort and risky.

I had a 78 year old patient come in a few years ago. He was suffering from knee pain, and the X-rays showed bone on bone in both knees. He had been a floor installer his entire life, crawling around on his hands and knees. His doctor had told him a bilateral knee replacement was his only option. He asked for my opinion. I explained that based on his age, I was concerned about the surgery because of the risks of complications and recovery time. I explained that he really had nothing to lose by doing therapy. If it helps, great. If it doesn't help, at least he would have better mobility and be in better shape, even if he ended up having the surgery. He decided to start therapy. Six weeks into therapy, all of his pain was gone. How could this be? He had bone on bone? The bone on bone was not changed. Wasn't the bone on bone the "cause" of the pain? Apparently not. Interestingly, many of the pain receptors are in the muscle tissues. Because the muscle dysfunction around his knees was the cause of the degeneration, by improving the muscle function, he gained overall function. The gain in function also lessened the stress on the knees and he didn't have symptoms anymore. This approach saved him time and money.

Not to mention he was able to avoid a potentially life threatening surgery. His Quality of Life is better, and he is actively doing the things he loves. Win. I have seen numerous similar situations over the years in practice. Shoulder, knee, hip, back, neck, wrist, and ankle degeneration that becomes asymptomatic with proper therapies.

ROADBLOCK #3
MISUNDERSTANDINGS

"It's not the things you think you know that get you into trouble, it is the things you know for sure, that are wrong, that get you into trouble."

Will Rogers

One of the biggest misunderstandings people have regarding reaching retirement with a fully functioning body and good Quality of life is Chiropractic care. Chiropractic is uniquely suited to be one of the largest contributors to keeping people moving and active throughout their lives. However, the common knowledge in the public is poor, and in fact, many of the ideas people have are simply false. I have spent over 27 years observing some of the crazy misunderstandings the public holds regarding Chiropractic care.

My Back Popped Out

The biggest misunderstanding people hold is that your back pops out of place. People believe this to mean that your spine dislocates, or pops out of joint, and a Chiropractor pops the vertebrae back into joint. This model has been know to be incorrect for a long time, however, many people still utilize it because of its simplicity. If you spend anytime in the gross anatomy lab, you realize that for a vertebra to pop out of the joint, it would take a significant trauma. When someone's back does pop out of place from trauma, that is called a facet dislocation. Facet dislocations are usually a very serious condition and typically requires surgical intervention to protect damage to the spinal cord. Most people with facet dislocations show up in the emergency room after a severe trauma with neurologic symptoms. This is not what chiropractors are treating day to day in their offices. Even in the beginning of Chiropractic, the term Subluxation was utilized, which means "less than a dislocation".

The use of this model has created many confusions in the healthcare world, and has hampered collaboration with other healthcare providers because the model just doesn't make sense to people trained in anatomy and physiology. This model has also created many confusions with the public and created false expectations in the delivery and outcomes of Chiropractic care.

I recently had a new patient come in for pain he was experiencing in his neck. The pain had been going on for months, and he had been taking over the counter medications, getting massages, and had been to several Chiropractors. One of the first things he said was, "I have been to six Chiropractors, and none of them have been able to pop my neck back in place!" My comment back to him was, "Well, we will be number seven, because your neck has not popped out of joint." He looked at me like I was crazy. This idea that his neck had "dislocated" created misunderstandings that then created unrealistic expectations in his mind. I asked him, "How many times have you gone to these Chiropractors?' You can guess his answer. He said, "Once, to each Chiropractor." After all, if your vertebrae is dislocated, how many times should you need to go to get it back "in place"? This misunderstanding created a whole list of negative feelings in his mind. He concluded that the Chiropractors were "no good," that Chiropractic "just didn't work," and that it was "a waste of his time and money." He was not happy.

So if your back is not popping out of place, what is happening?

As we have already discussed, joints have muscles that cross over the joint. In the spine, there are muscles that do the same. There are even deep small muscles, called stabilizer muscles, that cross over each vertebrae. When these small muscles get injured from things we do in life, the muscle contracts, shortens, and compresses the joint. This muscle contraction can also pull and compress the joint in different angles, depending on which muscles are involved. This gives the vertebrae the appearance of being out of alignment, because the vertebrae is out of alignment, NOT out of joint. Big difference. The mechanoreceptors in the joints, muscles, tendons, and skin are also signaling improperly.

When a Chiropractor does an adjustment to the vertebrae, the bones are being used as levers to stretch the deep muscle. When this stretching occurs rapidly, or with high velocity and amplitude, the muscles' mechanoreceptors are stimulated and a stretch reflex occurs, causing reflex relaxation of the muscles controlled by that motor unit. This reflex can also be stimulated through the mechanoreceptors with some of the instrument devices utilized in chiropractic. So really, the adjustment is done to the muscles, not the bone. And to refine it down even more, the adjustment is done to the mechanoreceptors in the muscles and tissues. This neurological event, even creates changes in the prefrontal cortex of the brain, potentially creating even more effects in the body that are still being researched today.

When these muscles reflexly relax, the joint decompresses. This takes pressure off the cartilage inside the joint, reducing the odds of developing arthritis. The relaxation of the muscle also restores the range of motion of the joint, which then prevents injury to the joint.

The vast majority of the patients I have seen over my career have been chronic cases. Chronic conditions are conditions that have been around for more than 12 weeks. Acute conditions are conditions that have happened suddenly and rapidly. Another category that isn't discussed much, is the acute exacerbation of a chronic condition. This is a chronic condition that flares up. There is much confusion in these areas. Much of the research done on back pain is acute back pain. This is interesting because I have rarely seen true acute conditions.

What I have seen mostly, is acute exacerbations of chronic conditions. I believe many doctors and therapists miss this diagnosis in the history of the patient. It is easy to do, as the patient in front of you is in severe pain. When you ask them when it happened, they say, "Two days ago." This gives the appearance of an acute injury. However, if you ask them, "Has this ever happened before?" They will typically say, "Yes, every month for the past ten years." Or, something similar showing that the symptom has happened before. This is not acute. This is an acute exacerbation of a chronic condition.

So, how do these deep muscles get hurt? The muscles get hurt from doing physical things in life. When you fall on the ice, but get up and feel ok. When you sit in the car for 12 hours, but just feel a little stiff. The hit you took in football, but you are fine. The rear end at 50 mph, but you didn't get hurt. The all day trip to the amusement park roller coaster rides, but you are fine. All these things in life can cause micro traumas that build up over time, like straw on the camel's back. Similar to repetitive strain injuries, like carpal tunnel, or neck pain from sitting at a desk for 20 years.

I was at a Chiropractic convention several years ago. All the Chiropractors were walking around looking at all the vendors and checking out the products at the booth. A lady Chiropractor walked past me and tripped on a cord running across the aisle. She caught herself and didn't fall, but was very close. I said, "Wow, that was a close one!" She said, "Yeah, but no big deal, if I fell one of the Chiropractors here could pop my back in joint." I observe these kinds of comments and conversations all the time. Not only from the public, but from healthcare providers, and even Chiropractors. Communicating how Chiropractic works is essential to developing understanding in the public, and value. This understanding is essential to help the public use less medications, have less arthritis, have fewer surgeries, and have a better overall Quality of Life!

Straw On The Camel's Back

As these seeming small injuries build up over time, you get stiffer and stiffer, and the joints get more compressed. As you asymptomatically lose ranges of motion, you are at more risk for injury. I call this the "Straw on the camel's back phenomena". Imagine if I had a camel here, and he could talk. I could put a piece of straw on his back, and ask him, "Did that hurt". He would say, "No." I could put more pieces of straw on his back and ask each time if it hurt him? He would say, "No." Eventually, I would put one more straw on his back and down he would go. He would then blame that last straw for causing his injury. When in reality, the cumulative load on his back is what caused the injury, and the last straw was simply the last straw. The cause was the cumulative load.

People are similar. Many of the patients I have seen over the years are unable to tell me how they got hurt. Or they will tell me something small and insignificant, blaming the last straw. For example, "I bent down to pick up a pencil and blew my back out". I always ask, "How much did the pencil weigh?" Obviously, not much. Think about this, if a 4 year old can pick up a pencil and not get hurt, a grown tough guy man should be able to do that without injury.

Here are some of the reasons patients have said caused their injury:

"I sneezed"

"I reached for my phone"

"The dog jumped on my lap"

"I picked up the shovel"

"I looked in my blind spot driving"

"The toaster popped and startled me"

"I hit a bump while driving"

"I slept wrong"

"I bent down to tie my shoe"

"I sat down on the toilet"

"I reached up to change a lightbulb"

"I put my seatbelt on"

Obviously, these and similar statements are just the last straw incident on a load they already carried, predisposing them to the injury.

In Grand Rapids, we have a really cool butterfly museum. You can walk through it, and literally hundreds of butterflies fly all around you and even land on you. Last year I had a patient come in and she couldn't move her neck. She was in severe pain. She had already been taking over the counter medications (OTC's), and had already been to the urgent care center to get prescription medications. She was still hurting after three months, and couldn't move, so she came into my clinic. When I asked her what she had done, she explained how she was at the butterfly museum. As she was walking around, she turned her head to see a butterfly, and her neck froze up. She blamed the butterfly. Clearly, the butterfly didn't hurt her, the movement was the last straw on the camel's back. But why? She likely already had a severe range of motion restrictions in her neck, even though she had no pain. The last straw was her turning to see the butterfly. So when did her problem begin? With the first straw, or the last? Imagine if I had tested her motion before she went to the butterfly museum. Likely, there would have been restrictions in her motion. We then found and corrected any range of motion restrictions, even though they were not symptomatic. Would she still have hurt her neck turning to look at the butterfly? I think not. The last straw is not the cause. Testing would likely have identified the problem before the butterfly incident.

Once you go to a chiropractor, you have to go forever

Have you ever heard anyone say, "Once you go, you have to go forever."? This statement prevents many people from seeking help at a Chiropractor. As I thought about this, I realized a few things. Why don't people say, "Don't go to the dentist, because once you go you have to go forever!"? Most people would consider that ridiculous. Or, how about don't go to the gym, because once you go you have to go forever?

This misunderstanding stems from thinking that your back pops out of joint and Chiropractors pop it back in joint. After all, that should just take one visit. Since Chiropractors are adjusting the receptors in the muscles, the muscles are what need to be changed.

By restoring range of motion and reducing muscle hypertonicity, the patient can reach better levels of movement. If you do not increase the patient's range of motion, yet they still feel better and quit care, they are just going to re-injure the area as soon as they do any activity that requires the restricted movement. They then go back to the Chiropractor because they are hurting again. This can happen over and over again. I call this the "Relief Care Cycle". Of course they will have the pain return if the cause is not changed. I would expect that to happen. This is what so many patients do, and have done for years. This is where the idea that "once you go you have to go forever" comes from. If a patient only seeks treatment when they have a symptom, they will likely experience the symptoms again unless the cause is corrected.

Seeing a Chiropractor because you have symptoms is different from seeing a Chiropractor to prevent injuries, prevent arthritis, and to have a better quality of life. While going for symptoms will likely create the "Relief Care Cycle," and you would end up "going forever" because the problem was never fixed. Going as a preventative measure would require you to "go forever" too. The difference is the purpose of the visit. Symptoms vs. prevention. Going in when you feel great is so you can be "checked out" to see if you have any areas of tension building up (straw on the camel's back) and have not yet produced symptoms. You can find these areas of build up by checking ranges of motion, palpating motion, palpating muscle tension and knots, utilizing technology like the Pro Adjuster, and using orthopedic testing. When this person arrives, they are there to be evaluated for restrictions in motion. The Chiropractor is treating the area of restricted motion. By restoring motion, there are less odds of injury, less odds of degeneration and arthritis, and better odds of being able to do the things you love to do!

Imagine if we cloned you. We had two of you. You #1 goes to the Chiropractor regularly, since childhood, even if you are not hurting. Anytime there is any tightness or tension building up, the Chiropractor finds and reduces the tension. After every bike crash, slide into third base, fall on the ice, hit in football, and all the other little "nothings" that we all do, you get checked. This keeps your joints mobile and allows you to be active with less buildup of "straw on your back". You #2 only goes to the Chiropractor when you are hurt and have symptoms. Play these two scenarios out until you are 75 years old. What do you think you would see? Who would move better? Who took fewer medications? Who was more hunchbacked?

Who would be more active? Who would be having a better overall Quality of Life? Not hard to figure out.

Limit the Odds of Success

All too often, I have observed people limiting their odds of success in reaching a functional retirement. They think that because they are doing one thing, that one thing is good enough. In order to have the best odds of success, you should do everything possible to help you in that endeavor. For example, a person who goes to the dentist and chiropractor regularly, eats healthy, takes supplements, drinks water, exercises, stretches, gets regular massages, avoids drugs, avoids smoking, and avoids alcohol will have better odds of success than someone who only does one of these things.

I was talking a few years ago with a guy at a health fair. I was explaining how Chiropractic could help him. His objection was that he didn't need Chiropractic because he took vitamins. He felt that was good enough. I gave him this example.

Imagine if your corvette was starting to pull to one side when you were driving. You noticed that one tire was wearing out more. So, you decided to head over to the gas station. When you pulled up to the pumps, you picked the premium fuel pump. You filled up with expensive gas. Would that fix your alignment problem? Unlikely. Even though you were doing something good, that doesn't mean it addresses all issues. Just like if a person only does Chiropractic care, but eats at McDonalds everyday, they will still likely have problems.

I stumbled upon this idea of "odds of success" back in the early 2000's. Fibromyalgia was a big problem for a lot of people, and there were really no conventional medical treatments. Many medical providers wouldn't even consider fibromyalgia a real disease or condition. In fact, many patients were being told that the symptoms of fibromyalgia were "all in their head". This caused many patients to seek out alternative methods of help. We saw a huge influx of patients with the symptoms of fibromyalgia.

After treating hundreds of patients, I started to notice some patterns. One of the big things I noticed was patients were trying all sorts of treatments. Vitamins, Physical Therapy (PT), Chiro, Massage, yoga, exercise, stretching, water aerobics, etc. I frequently saw patients who had tried numerous different therapies. One thing they didn't do, was to do all these different therapies together. When we started to put multiple therapies together, we started to see major breakthroughs for patients. For example, a lady came in who had tried Physical Therapy, but it didn't work. She tried Chiropractic, but it didn't work. She took vitamins, but it didn't work. She exercised, but it didn't work. She changed her diet, but it didn't work. So, I asked her, "What do you mean by 'didn't work'?" She said, "I didn't feel better." The first thing I had to tackle was her concept of results. She had no measurements other than her symptoms. As we completed her exam, we now had a good baseline of her function, in addition to her symptoms. The next step was to address her mindset of combining therapies. She was told by her Physical Therapist to only do one therapy at a time. That way she would know which therapy worked. The problem with this approach is that often each therapy will help a little bit, but not always enough to notice symptomatic improvement. However, by combining therapies, the cumulative effects could happen, and results were more likely to occur. The different therapies are working on different muscles, tissues, receptors, joints, nerves, etc. By approaching the patient holistically, we were able to see major improvements in function, measured by improvements in range of motion, balance, muscle hypertonicity, muscle knots, and strength. This combination of therapies became a huge success for many fibromyalgia patients. Once their function started to improve, the patients would start to feel better. This took time. By routinely measuring function, we could see if we were making improvements, even if the patient wasn't feeling better yet. Some patients had great functional improvements, even if their symptoms changes were less dramatic. However, the patient's quality of life was always better when they had better function. I coined the saying, "You never lose when your function improves". Improved function is what keeps you able to do all the things you want to do today, and in your retirement. The secret was combining therapies, measuring improvements, and educating the patients so they would understand and follow through to obtain results. The more positive things you can do, the better your odds of success.

Another common reason people would tell me that they don't need a Chiropractor was because they work out. Somehow, Chiropractic was just for "out of shape" people. This was weird to me, as virtually every elite athlete was utilizing Chiropractic care to improve performance and rehabilitate injuries. Arnold, Tiger, Venus, Brady, and many other elites, to name a few. What people don't think about, is that sports and life is literally a "Game of Inches". Your mobility will determine your performance. If you are tight and stiff, you will likely perform poorly, and be more likely to get injured.

I had a baseball pitcher come into the office a few years ago. He felt fine and didn't think he needed any treatments. Upon examination, I found his pitching shoulder had an asymptomatic restriction in motion. I asked him if he thought the restriction was helping or hurting his performance. He agreed it probably wasn't helping. After treating his shoulder, he regained full range of motion. He pitched the following weekend in a tournament. When he came back he explained how he threw over 90 mph the whole tournament, which he had never done before. Range of motion matters. A little tightness could be the difference between hitting a homer or a strike out, a golf ball in the woods or on the green, a volleyball landing in or out. It always comes down to one thing. How well a person actually understands the value Chiropractic delivers, and the common sense principles. The problem is, very few people do understand. When you don't understand, you don't value. When you don't value, you don't do. When you don't do it, you don't get results.

"I Already Know"

Another misunderstanding I have encountered is people thinking they "already know" all about chiropractic. This is interesting, as most people know very little, and what they do know is incorrect. In fact, you could write a book about all the misunderstandings, LOL. Think about it, when you think you know, you don't listen. You shut down. Learning does not occur. I have found many patients can't learn because they think they already know.

The "I Already Know" phenomenon happens in all areas of life. Really, what "I Already Know" means, is that you have already DECIDED what you think about a topic. In life, we all have so many decisions to make that it can be overwhelming. Once we make a decision about how we think or feel about something, that decision gets put into the file cabinet in your mind and doesn't allow any new information. It is the DECIDED file. In fact, any new information that is contrary to the decision we made is protectively dismissed so we are not wrong. Any data that is consistent with our decision is allowed, as that reinforces the decision we made. This holds true in so many areas from religion, politics, health, and really all subjects. Life is easier this way, which is why people do this. The DECIDED file can be made by our own experiences, stories we hear from others, media, and really anything/anyone that the person holds as a trusted source of information.

A few weeks ago a new patient came in to my office. She had back pain, and has been to Chiropractors for 30 years. As I did her exam, she kept interrupting and telling me to just crack her back. That she didn't need an exam, she knew what she needed. She explained that she knew everything about Chiropractic because she has been going for decades, and her brother was a Chiropractor. Interesting. She explained that she knows when she needs it because she hurts. When her back first hurt, it would only take a visit or two and she was "fine". Now, it typically takes several adjustments before her back feels better. Her reasoning was because Chiropractors are not as good as they used to be. She has been doing symptom based care (Relief Care) for decades, experiencing the Relief Care Cycle, and gradually getting worse and degenerating more and more. She went on to explain how her symptomatic condition has been getting worse over the years. Shocker. This is from a patient who "knows all about it". As we talked, and I explained more, she started to realize that she had made some poor choices (Relief Care) with bad outcomes (Degeneration/Arthritis). She didn't understand the importance of testing to determine dysfunction. She only understood the symptoms. Just because someone knows how to lay on a table and get adjusted, does not mean they understand how things work and how to get the best results, even if her brother is a Chiropractor. In fact, she understood very little, and required a lot of communication to open up her DECIDED mind.

My Mom used to cut hair when I was growing up. She had a salon in our house, and people would come over to get their hair cut, colored, permed, or whatever. I watched her do thousands of haircuts over the years. I have experienced many haircuts myself. I know it doesn't look like it, LOL. Yet, that experience does not mean I know all about cutting hair. Just because my Mom is a hairdresser, does not mean you want me to cut your hair.

The best way to cut through the mindset of someone who "Already Knows," is to just ask them simple questions. When they don't know the answers, they tend to realize that they don't know, and they are more likely to open their DECIDED file and learn. Not everyone is able to open the DECIDED file, as it is too painful for them to be wrong. Helping people to make some new decisions that are seemingly unrelated to what they already have in the DECIDED file can often help open the DECIDED file. When they see that they have two decisions in the DECIDED file that are not congruent will allow some to reevaluate all of the evidence and make a new decision to put in the DECIDED file. Some good questions are:

How do I know where to adjust you? Answer, the testing.

How do you know when you need to be adjusted? Answer, the testing.

How do I know how often to recommend you get adjusted? Answer, the testing.

What does an adjustment do? It causes a quick stretch on the deep stabilizer muscles which causes a stretch reflex and the muscles relax around the joint which decompresses the joint and causes stimulation to the prefrontal cortex.

What is the cracking and popping noise with manual adjustments? Answer, cavitation. When the adjustment relaxes the muscles, the joint opens rapidly, the liquid in the joint turns to gas rapidly which gives off energy causing the cracking noise.

Why does it take more than one adjustment? Answer: Muscles need frequency to change. You can't just stretch or workout one time and think you will be good. There is a term called muscle CREEP. Creep is where the muscle will pull back to how it was prior to the treatment. After each treatment, there is less creep, until ideally the muscle is back to normal function.

I try hard to be open minded and realize that new things are discovered every day. The minute you think you know it all, is the minute you are disconnected from becoming better. Change the name of your DECIDED file. Rename it OPEN TO MORE DATA file.

Fear

Fear is another excuse. In fact, I believe the number one reason people don't go to a Chiropractor is because they are afraid of being twisted and turned. What people don't realize, is that adjustments are very safe. While everything in life has risks, adjustments have been shown to be safer than taking aspirin. Most people don't think twice about taking aspirin. Much of the fear comes from lack of understanding. When you don't understand something, it can be scary. If you haven't experienced something, it can be scary. I have had thousands of conversations with people who are afraid of getting adjusted and of Chiropractors in general. Alleviating their concerns to the level of acceptance has a low probability of success. While I have convinced many, it certainly hasn't been most. What I have found to be very effective, is instead of arguing with them, just change the concept. Move the conversation to the computerized adjustment. The Pro Adjuster is one of the tools I utilize in my offices. When you show this instrument to a potential patient, it is astonishing how their fears will be put to rest. There is no twisting and turning. The computer detects where the vertebrae are not moving properly, from the deep stabilizer muscles being hypertonic or dysfunctional. The computer can then stimulate the mechanoreceptors in these muscles and cause a reflex relaxation of the muscles. This restores the vertebral motion, and patients will then start to feel better.

Some people say they had a bad experience with a Chiropractor. This can be for a million different reasons. The best approach is to simply explain it this way:

Have you ever had a bad haircut? Yes. Did you never get a haircut again, as the profession is bad, or did you just go to another barber/hairdresser?

Have you ever had a bad server at a restaurant? Did you never go out to eat again because the profession of servers is bad? Or did you realize it was just that experience and you went out to eat again?

Realize that there is good and bad in every profession, and in every experience. We all have good days and bad days. Help people see that they need to have a little grace.

Some patients have come in over the years who say that they were hurt by a Chiropractor. They DECIDED that the profession hurt them, and would never go to another Chiropractor. After talking with them, I have found that about 95% of the people I spoke with who said they were hurt meant they were sore. After all, the word "hurt" can mean many different things to people.

The vast majority of the people who told me they were hurt by a Chiropractor have a story similar to Jennifer's story.

I met Jennifer at a health expo. She decided to stop at my booth and tell me how a Chiropractor she went to five years ago had hurt her. After she told her story, I asked her a few questions.

Me: "How many times did you go to this Chiropractor?"

Jennifer: "The one time"

Me: "What did you feel when you were hurt?"

Jennifer: "The next day my neck was super sore for two days and I had headaches."

Me: "Wow, sorry to hear that!" "Did the Dr. tell you that you could feel that way after the treatment?"

Jennifer: "No."

Me: "Did you go back?"

Jennifer: "No way!"

Me: "What do you think happened?"

Jennifer: "He wrenched on my neck and popped it out of place more."

Me: "Were you under the impression that one treatment would fix your neck problem?"

Jennifer: "Well, yeah, it needed to be popped back in place."

Me: "I believe I understand what happened." Would you like to know?"

Jennifer: "Yes."

Me: "Have you ever been to the gym?"

Jennifer: "Yes"

Me: "If your muscles are out of shape, how do you feel the next day?"

Jennifer: "Sore"

Me: "Right, the gym wasn't bad and hurt you, your muscles just were not used to movement and you were sore, but it is what you needed." "Since the adjustments are to your muscles, not your bones popping out of place, and those muscles are not in shape. How do you think those muscles are going to feel after a treatment?"

Jennifer: "Sore...I wished they would have told me that!"

As you can see, understanding is critical for patients to achieve results. You can diagnose Jennifer's misunderstandings by the comments she made. This allows you to help by explaining more in depth, so she can make an informed decision.

SO NOW WHAT
DO YOU DO?

"When your function improves, you never lose."

Dr. Michael Kwast

N ow that you have discovered the importance of staying mobile, here are some ideas to get you started.

#1 Find a chiropractor who will measure your ranges of motion, perform orthopedic testing, perform functional movement testing, and keep you informed of your inabilities, even if you are not symptomatic. These motions include orthopedic, functional movements, and spinal range of motion, individual spinal segmental range of motion, and extremity joints' ranges of motion. These movements are essential to keep moving and lowering your chances of injury and degenerative arthritis. Your movement restrictions are what you are treating, NOT just your symptoms. If the Chiropractor doesn't understand, find another one. Also, incorporate a massage therapist into your treatments. When the massage therapist is aware of your movement restrictions, they can focus on restoring those motions. Instead of just a relaxing massage, functional restoration is the key. When the chiropractor and massage therapist are both aware of your physical limitations, the goal becomes fixing the limitations, not just working on what hurts. This can be confusing for many, as most therapy is built around your symptoms. Keep focused on WHY you are doing these therapies. You are doing them to keep your ranges of motion! Don't fall into the trap of thinking it is about how you feel at the moment.

#2 Get a sleep study. Many dentists will provide this service, as well as medical physicians. When sleep problems are detected early, there are often effective options available besides just a c-pap. Oral appliances can be very effective to open your airways while sleeping. When you are not getting effective sleep, you are setting yourself up for disaster. Some of the research shows poor sleep can take up to ten years off of your life! If you are always tired, and/or snore, this is very likely significant.

#3 Get some screenings from companies like lifeline. They can ultrasound your arteries, do an EKG of your heart, check blood work, and other tests to determine where potential problems may be lurking asymptomatically.

#4 Get on some good multivitamins. Have your Chiropractor help you figure out what you should be taking.

#5 Eat healthy. This is probably not what you think. There is a lot of misinformation out there regarding diet. So many people say they are "vegan," yet eat a dozen donuts a day. You are probably eating too many carbs, too much sugar, and too many processed foods. The easiest way to cut through all the details, is to simply eat food the way it is found in nature. This means fruits, vegetables, fish, and meat. The less processed the better. The fewer hormones and antibiotics the better.

#6 Get outside and get some sunshine. Sunlight helps with melatonin levels, which regulates your sleep and moods. Sunlight on your skin also allows your body to make vitamin D, which is essential for good body function.

#7 Start exercising and stretching. Based on your movement examination, the chiropractor should be able to give you a list of exercises and stretches to help improve your mobility. Remember, the goal is your ability to move. You are probably not competing in the olympics. Bicep curls and running for miles is probably not what you need to be doing. Functional movements are things you need to do in everyday life. Do exercises like, go up and down the stairs 20 times, lay down on the floor and get back up 20 times, squat down on your heels 20 times, crawl on the carpet and get back up 20 times, do pull-ups.

If you need help, hire a personal trainer. Make sure they understand your functional movement goals and range of motion limitations, so they can set up an effective program.

#8 Start balance therapy proactively. Balance is a big problem for the elderly, and falls are a major cause of nursing home admissions. Your Chiropractor and trainer can help you with a program. You can also get a balance board for home-work. Practice standing on one leg, and as you become more advanced, practice standing on one leg with your eyes closed.

Anything you can do now to increase your mobility and function is a win. No one gets less stiff over time. As we age, we are all moving towards the ultimate stiffness of rigor mortis! The key is to understand and implement the strategies I have outlined. When you do this, you will give yourself the best odds of success of having a better quality of life today, and into your retirement. Don't end up sitting in a rocking chair and paying bills. Implement your retirement plan financially and physically. Live your best quality of life by staying active and mobile. And as the Soup Nazi from Seinfeld would say if he wrote this, "No rocking chair for you!"